The A-Z companion guide to orthopaedic surgery

The A-Z companion guide to orthopaedic surgery

An essential reference book to support those undergoing the inconvenience and frustrations of their orthopaedic surgery

Chris Maslin

FIRST EDITION

ISBNs:

978-1-80541-042-3 (paperback)

978-1-80541-043-0 (eBook)

Foreword

I have lived with osteoarthritis for over 10 years and, having undergone a total hip replacement operation at the perceived early age of fifty-three, I wish that I had known in advance what lay ahead of me before, during and indeed after the operation.

Our NHS continues to perform wonders in the most difficult of circumstances and their pre-operative and post-operative literature provides an extremely helpful insight into the operation. This does not, however, focus so much on the anxiety of the patient and some of the more obscure, embarrassing and practical daily obstacles faced afterwards.

Realistically, everyone knows of an elderly friend or relative who has undergone a successful knee replacement or hip operation. The experience is not any less daunting or traumatic for the individual concerned, who may be experiencing this procedure for the very first time.

The content of this reference guide should not be construed as medical advice, but it will show you that you are not alone with any fears or concerns that you may have. It's designed to provide you with helpful tips and suggestions to support your mental health and aid your recovery.

With certainty, readers will be in a position to avoid some of the schoolboy errors that I made during the experience. Friends and family may also be able to use this information to increase their personal awareness and support of a loved one after they have faced the inconvenience and embarrassment of such a major operation.

Index

Anaesthetic

————◆————

I was invited to attend the hospital for my operation at 07:30 on the day, but I was not called for surgery until late afternoon. I had incorrectly assumed that it would take place in the morning, so I would definitely recommend taking a book to read.

Be prepared for a long wait as I understand the rota is only agreed in the morning, although the hospital staff do provide water to patients in this position. This is understandably withdrawn three hours before the operation, in line with your advised fasting guidelines.

One tip I learnt is not to sit facing the nurses during the "dry" period as it's exceedingly difficult to watch staff taking large swigs from their water bottles, especially when you are understandably nervous and your mouth is so dry.

The anaesthetist will meet with you to discuss the procedure and it was very reassuring to watch a heavy black marker pen being used to draw a clear arrow on my affected limb. This dispelled my previous nightmares that I would awaken from the operation to find that my perfect hip was now radically altered.

Many of you who suffer from osteoarthritis will know that putting on lower clothes is extremely difficult and, rather ashamedly, I did issue an expletive when a nurse asked me to prepare for the operation by putting on a pair of hospital-issue brown socks and white underpants.

Not only did I think the colour scheme was back to front, but I did find this hard to digest, as the main reason for being there was to address my restricted

movement. These garments had miraculously disappeared after the operation, so answers on a postcard
are most welcome as to their purpose.

The best advice I can give you is to listen carefully to
what is said by the anaesthetist(s) and to allow the
experts to work their magic in preparation for your
operation, as it will soon be over.

Bottle

———◆———

One of my first recollections of being introduced to my hospital bed after the operation was observing a "cardboard sock" on my tray and I subsequently thought it was a carafe of wine; a genuinely nice and unexpected gesture from the surgeon, I thought.

Several frantic text messages to my friends later and I was quickly made to realise this was in fact my pee bottle. However, in my implausible defence, there were no instructions on the front.

Readers will be pleased to know that I have not researched a similar bottle for women, but I guess it's a rather similar device. I am not necessarily advocating that you practice with one in advance, but this will hopefully make you more aware than I was of what may need to be done.

Once I had mastered the intellectual challenge of how to use this device, I recall how relieved I was (excuse the pun) once I had accomplished my task. I used to feel so very smug that I called the nurse immediately to replenish the stocks and take away the empties; in all fairness, there is very little else for you to do.

Should you need a device or bottle at home during the early stages of recovery, then I would strongly urge you to store the bottle in a warm place beforehand. From personal experience, it certainly does focus your mind when you try and use a bottle which is freezing cold.

Commando

———◆———

A lot has been packed into my 54th year on this planet as, in addition to writing several books and using a pee bottle for the first time, I also gained my first experience of going commando and not wearing underwear.

I initially thought how wrong this was but the last thing you want after the operation is to provide yourself with further dressing problems and trip hazards, so underwear took a back seat for the first 4 weeks of my recovery.

The advice I had received was to bring lounge clothes for wearing on the ward and I remember packing three entire changes of clothes, plus those which I had worn on the day of the operation. Hindsight tells me this was a little excessive for a 3-night stay!

I had treated myself to Rupert Bear-type pyjama bottoms and T-shirts, which I lived in post-operatively for much longer than I should probably admit to. I would strongly advocate that you pack loungewear only, as comfort is your absolute priority.

Whilst I spent a lot of time in bare feet, please also be very careful with footwear. Proudly remembering my lightweight shoes, I made a big mistake in not realising that my size 10 feet would subsequently grow into size 12, with the post-operative swelling.

The result was an enormous water blister and several visits to my local GP. In all honesty I could have done without this, considering my post-operative mobility issues.

Dressing

———◆———

A welcome addition to your "hospital takeaway kit" (please read on) should be a sock-aid and shoehorn and these both took some getting used to.

Whilst there are plenty of videos on YouTube covering the subject of putting on socks post-operatively, it's not quite as easy as it sounds.

For the early part of my recovery, socks went the same way as underwear as barefoot seemed quite sensible; not so good for when you wish to start walking and exercising.

Throughout the recovery process, I was paranoid about exceeding a 90-degree hip rotation and I was determined not to risk anything.

I was lucky enough to receive assistance with pulling up trousers and putting on socks and this was necessary due to the bending restrictions mentioned above. However, if you are not so fortunate and do not have assistance, then I would suggest acquiring cheap aids to practice with in advance.

Once you have mastered the art of putting your socks on, and despite this sounding silly, please don't forget to practice taking your socks off. This action requires a different stretch of the muscles entirely and it's very easy to keep them on for several days if you find this difficult in the preliminary stages of your recovery.

Exercise and Stairs

———◆———

I had received advanced notification from the hospital of the exercises that I would need to do and these involved moving my leg forwards, backwards and sideways (never crossways) and it had been suggested that I practice these in advance.

Although initially sceptical, I now fully endorse these exercises as you may find they are not so easy as they first appear, immediately after your operation.

Nurses will try and get you on your feet as soon as possible (often the same day) and you will rapidly become acquainted with a Zimmer frame and crutches. The crutches were an entirely new concept to me and, when using one crutch, this should be used on the side of the non-affected joint.

To be released from hospital, you will have to show the hospital physio that you can ascend / descend the specially constructed hospital stairs. These are often far less severe than the ones you may usually be faced with and I would emphasise that you should take great care when you first attempt stairs at home.

The mnemonic is "Good leg to heaven" and "Bad leg to hell" when you work out which leg to lead with. This is translated as good leg first when you ascend, bad leg first when you descend. Bannisters are crucial and it's particularly important that you are escorted when using stairs initially, until you feel confident with doing this on your own.

Walking is quite rightly considered the fundamental exercise for recovery. Not only does this help build your confidence, but it's also a great conversation-starter for when you are outside and walking in some initial discomfort; beware of large and friendly dogs though.

Friends

——◆——

This is a wonderful opportunity to evaluate your friends and support network as you really do need those close to you to come up trumps.

It's amazing how much difference a phone call or a simple cup of coffee with a friend can make to improving your day.

Many of you will know someone who has been through a similar experience and you can learn from them what works and what doesn't. Initially, you will soon go stir crazy and there is only so much television you can manage. You will also be in some discomfort and on medication so it's certainly worth taking some time beforehand to work out how you will cope.

Should you be on your own, then make this known to your hospital in advance so they can undertake a risk assessment, remembering that food preparation and meal provision cannot be taken for granted.

Beware of friends who are not the greatest thinkers before they speak! Shortly after my operation, I vividly remember one acquaintance telling me that it "only" took a year for her brother to recover from a similar operation; yeah, thanks.

Without hesitation, I know that I will be there in a flash for any of my friends who helped me through this ordeal and they will always remain a very important part of my life.

Grabber

——◆——

Another big thank you goes to our NHS for this fantastic item.

I had grown quite attached to my grabber and it was especially useful for picking up dropped items and assisting with dressing from the waist down.

When you are very bored, it can also imitate a gun. You can then point this at the screen whenever annoying politicians or news reporters appear on your telly.

There are various gadgets which can be attached to the grabber to enable you to hang things from, and further included is a wonderful plastic end. This serves very well to soothe that most annoying of itches, although I am not sure that's exactly what it's designed for.

With practice and patience, this tool can be most useful in assisting you with your recovery, apart from when you leave it downstairs after going to bed. Upon reflection, two of these wonderful tools would have been a very good idea.

Highs and Lows

I found the build-up to my operation incredibly stressful as not only was there every chance that it may be cancelled, given the climate that we currently live in, but I also knew that I should have been losing weight to speed up the recovery.

I could easily have challenged how I could have been expected to achieve this with my restricted mobility and limping, but comfort binge eating certainly did not help me in the long run.

There will be many ups and downs along the way but it's important to focus on the end result and the feeling of inner joy when you manage to stand, fully weight-bearing, on your operated leg again for the first time.

Instantly, the pain in my hip disappeared and each slight improvement greatly improved my mental health. Before you know it, you will no longer have any excuse for lounging around watching telly all day.

What drove me to write this book was the need to access further information during my recovery and, should you google the subject enough, you will find there are lots of tips and forums out there.

Subject matter is written by people who have successfully undergone exactly the same operations and experiences as you and I and participating on these forums can provide you with a truly wonderful sense of community and belonging.

Irritations

As you undergo your recovery, there will be many niggles along the way. In my innocence, I was consumed by the inner belief and understanding that 4-6 weeks is the average time for you to completely return to normal; this is a fallacy.

This period of time is a good benchmark for resuming many activities and movements that you were used to doing, but please do not be fooled into believing that you will be in full working order on Day 43.

Everybody will hear a story about Aunty Gladys who managed to leap around within two weeks of surgery but please listen to your own body and do what feels right for you.

Following my 6-week check-up, I received a positive evaluation from my surgeon and indeed he informed me that I could drive again. I was especially pleased when my car decided to start right away but I quickly decided that I didn't feel confident in resuming driving so quickly. My attention was not focused on looking ahead as it was still directed far too much towards my wound.

I also suffered from pain in the back, groin and heel but was pleased to learn that these were common post-operative ailments. It's always reassuring to know that you are not alone when you experience these, although they are irritating when they impact your sleep and comfort.

Remind yourself repeatedly of your end game and it's amazing how quickly the body will repair itself. Friends have even commented on how much taller I am, now that I am no longer hampered by a limp and leaning to one side.

Jewellery

———◆———

Many hospitals do not provide you with secure lockers or safety deposit boxes for valuables and, whilst you are otherwise engaged during surgery, your belongings may be handled by several other people who are unaware of your individual possessions or hospital ward number.

Therefore, I would suggest that you give this matter some thought when it comes to bringing any valuable personal items with you.

Post-operatively, you are not going to be especially worried about looking pristine and you may also be too groggy to know where you have stored things. It may therefore be a better idea to leave said valuables with family or a close friend who can return these to you once you are back in the real world.

With hindsight, I would have only taken my phone (and charger) as when you are discharged, the adrenalin and sense of excitement means you are in such a rush to leave the hospital before they change their mind. You may not be concentrating on where you have stored these items, leading to the inconvenience of a search that both you and the hospital staff can easily do without.

Kitchen

———◆———

For those of you who are facing recovery on your own, it's worth spending a considerable amount of time planning for your return.

Suddenly, many cupboards and drawers may no longer be within your reach and I would strongly advocate a good supply of accessible ready meals for the first couple of weeks after you return home.

I remember feeling very pleased with myself that I had made a coffee, using my crutches for support, until I realised that I had to make the return journey to my chair. Upon reflection, the kettle should perhaps have been relocated too.

The hospital will, I am certain, make sure that you receive assistance where needed and this is where friends can step in once more.

Home deliveries are more common these days but that's not particularly helpful when you are reliant on your grabber to pick up and store your groceries; advance preparation is key.

Lavatory

After my initial problems with a bottle, I confess that I was dreading this and I soon quickly realised why the hospital advises you to empty your bowels in advance of the operation. This is probably not the only reason but one that stands out.

Luckily, there is the most wonderful of inventions called a raised toilet seat and I would advise those of you who are having a hip operation to check with the hospital whether you can borrow one for home use if needed, as you really don't want to sit lower or bend more than you have to.

The hospital toilet also has rails for you to cling on to for dear life and when I got home, I got into a routine of using a Zimmer to assist me both onto and off from the toilet seat. Hopefully, your medications will distract you from how ridiculous you may look.

As your recovery progresses, this does without doubt get easier and some of the medications are known to have side effects that may cause constipation, which I was quite happy to have in the first couple of days.

When I knew that I could not put it off any longer, I informed the nurse of where I was going and, some 20 minutes later, I returned exhausted and was greeted with a wonderful and knowing smile from the nurse. On your first toilet visit, you may wish to consider taking a magazine with you to read and you may even have enough time for a cup of tea.

Medications

Naturally, the prescribing of your meds will depend on your individual circumstances and specifically tailored medical advice, but I was surprised that I did not rattle after the first couple of days.

One tip I quickly learnt was to make a note of when I would be given the meds in hospital so that I could try and nap around them, as sometimes I had just dropped off as the nurses were doing their rounds.

Upon discharge, you will rival a chemist with the supplies that you are provided with. However, the discharge nurse very helpfully labelled the meds and noted down their associated dosages and times for when I got home.

Whilst you will get into a routine as time passes by, it's very important to make sure that you take your medication at the right time and manage your pain relief; you may wish to ask a friend to help you with a timetable you can refer to.

I also made sure that any spare meds were kept upstairs where possible as I learnt quickly that you really do not want to have to get up and retrieve painkillers from downstairs in the middle of the night.

Nurses

A lot has quite rightly been written about what a wonderful job the NHS and nurses continue to do in this most difficult of times. My experience was no exception, particularly during the Covid pandemic.

I often felt guilty pressing the call button whilst the nurses set about their duties, but each time I was greeted efficiently, politely and made to feel like an individual rather than a number.

Please remember there are a huge number of people waiting for exactly the same operation as you, so try to focus on being grateful and treating each and every one of the staff with the respect and dignity they deserve.

There is also no place for modesty in the hip region and, for those more bashful readers, please don't let it worry you. The nurses have more than likely seen it all before and you will be more relieved at having your wound checked than facing the perceived embarrassment of dropping your trousers.

Within a fortnight, I needed to have my staples out and I remember being quite worried about this in advance, but it sounds worse than it actually is. Whilst you may resemble a piece of paper having a staple extractor applied to it, think of something nice and remember that you've had a lot worse done to you quite recently.

Operation

Naivety about my procedure enabled me to become a victim of pre-operative gags from my "friends" along the lines of having my leg raised behind my ear during the operation.

However, the hospital will provide literature and video links to demonstrate what happens during the operation. Being of a squeamish nature, I gave these a fairly wide berth as I wanted to give myself an outside chance of turning up on the day.

I also performed incredibly badly in science and biology at school and this is another reason for me to suggest that you leave specific medical advice concerning your condition to medical professionals.

What I would suggest, however, is to be careful when clicking on YouTube as this often provides more information than you would be comfortable with knowing. I can tell by my scar exactly where the surgeon has been and that is plenty of knowledge for me on the subject, thank you.

Pre-op

I found very little information as to what checks would be done before the operation and incorrectly assumed that it would just be height and weight.

Not knowing what lay ahead didn't help my blood pressure reading and this had to be retaken later during the appointment.

Please also be prepared for several tests including a blood sample, ECG (note to men – shave chest first) and groin swab – yes, that one caught me unawares.

There was an opportunity to ask questions at the end of the assessment so I would suggest a little prep time in advance to write down any queries that you may still have. You may also find out the scheduled date for your operation after they have performed your tests.

Without a doubt, it all felt very real after this visit and it's at this point that your preparations should well and truly begin.

Questions

In addition to your opportunity to ask questions at the pre-op, you will also have the chance to speak to your surgeon (or team member) post-operatively and this will probably be after six weeks.

Your journey until this point will have been quite a challenge and I would encourage you to jot down questions or concerns as you go along; you can always delete some of these should they no longer apply.

The last thing you want to do is to kick yourself (not easy) for not asking something that has been bugging you, when given your best opportunity to find out the answer.

When I saw the surgeon, I had 16 questions and I admit that I nicked some of these from the internet.

When you may resume driving is one of the most common questions asked at this time, but I also used the opportunity to have my wound checked and seek an opinion concerning some ongoing aches and pains. It was also reassuring to have the surgeon watch me walk again, with and without a crutch.

Rest

———◆———

However silly it sounds, you may find yourself easily exhausted as your recovery progresses. The uneducated and unaware may fail to grasp this; after all, how difficult can it be sleeping and sitting in a chair watching television? Let me answer that – very!

I downloaded the entire box set of Game of Thrones for my recovery and I was so distracted and dozy that I struggled to recall more than one character from the show, let alone the names of the dragons.

Should you find yourself dropping off, then allow yourself to do so, hopefully remembering to put down your cup of tea first. In the early days, this will allow for any remaining anaesthetic to clear from your system.

Please remember that the mental anxiety will take its toll on your recovery and you are likely to feel tired at many unconventional times of the day.

Sleeping

———•———

Here, you have a fantastic opportunity to become accustomed to another great piece of kit – the leg-up device. The idea is to hook up your leg onto the bed to minimise bending and, as with other hospital gadgets referred to in this guide, practice beforehand may indeed be a clever idea.

For the first 6 weeks after the operation, it was recommended that I sleep on my back with a towel between my legs and this was a struggle as I had always previously slept on my front or side.

Referred pain in the back and groin didn't help me with lying flat and I was initially quite fearful of nights.

In hindsight, I wish that I had become accustomed to sleeping on my back prior to my operation.

Whilst you will also nap during the day, it's important that you resume as close to your normal sleeping pattern as you can as quickly as possible.

Toiletries

———•———

I packed cheap and smaller versions of my essentials to reduce space in my bag and the embarrassing memory I have is of trying to shave on my third day.

The stubble would not shift for love or money and the nurse kindly supplied me with a new disposable razor. It was only when I returned home that I realised that I had not removed the plastic cap from my own device.

During the first 48 hours, I was not consumed with undue concerns over my body odour, but I was surprised how quickly that changed. You soon become conscious of your appearance to others, especially when you are on your feet and seeing the physio and doctor.

Without doubt, you need a lift during the early days. You may wish to give this matter some prior consideration to help you ease your journey away from the culture and habits of hospital life and back to some form of normality at home.

Uncertainty

———•———

I cannot stress enough the impact that the build-up to your operation can have on your mental health.

Granted, you have probably lived with the condition for a number of years. As the day approaches it's very hard not to become distracted, until your name is called.

Please remember that whilst many of these operations are referred to as major surgery, they are indeed also routine and increasingly commonplace.

With the greatest planning and hopefully using some of the advice contained in this guide, I am sure you will agree it really is a wonderful opportunity to improve your life.

Leading up to my operation, I spoke to a few acquaintances in my village about their experiences and just hearing about their successes really improved the mindset.

Vision

———•———

It may seem an odd title for this chapter but the other idea I had was Valium and I thought it may impact the sales of my book as I didn't want to be confused with a medical directory. Fear not, there is also more logic so please read on.

Knowing that I also suffer increasingly from OCD as my years continue to roll on by, I used to foresee what lay ahead when I was having my darkest moments during my recovery.

After learning to cope with early problems such as pain, mobility, and dressing, I then soon replaced these with positive thoughts as to how my situation would improve the following week.

Once I had achieved small milestones, such as moving from two crutches to one, I also used to reminisce on how difficult things had been during the previous weeks. I used every small win to project myself forward and to focus on how soon it would be until I could once again walk unaided.

Wound

————◆————

Initially, the post-operative dressing was in place for around two weeks, and I admit to letting my wound irritate me more than it should have. The nurses would check it until my release, but after that you are advised to seek medical assistance should it become spongy; let the paranoia begin.

After the first two weeks my dressing was changed and, despite being told my scar was now healed, I was advised not to remove my new dressing for another fortnight.

Removing the dressing scared me, to be honest, and I called in a favour from a medical friend who kindly did this for me. I repaid them with a bottle of wine so they could drink away the memory.

Depending on the season in which you have the operation, you may also wish to consider wearing shorts or clothing that does not rub, thus avoiding additional discomfort and irritation. What does improve the situation, however, is when you are able to sleep on your non-operated side once the wound has healed.

X-Ray

————◆————

After the operation, you are taken for an X-ray and I nervously asked my physio whether I could see the results. Once I had seen them, I realised the operation had been a success.

From suffering the agony of bone on bone, I could now see a clear gap which reflected the absence of the throbbing pain I had felt and I allowed myself a sneaky peek at my other hip. I was pleased for my untrained eye to observe that it still had some life about it yet.

The subsequent consultation also meant that I did not require a further X-ray, which was good to know from the length of appointment and parking meter perspective.

Without a doubt, my positivity increased from here and I started to realise that it had all been worth it.

Yesterday

Initially, all days will appear the same and you will be suffering from acute inertia in the early days of recovery.

Some days, I would awake to reflect on the day before and I soon realised this was a mistake; yesterday's events should be left just there – in the past.

To this day, I often reproach myself for how badly I behaved towards loved ones during my recovery, not realising or accepting the impact the operation had on me.

Whilst it's understandable to feel sorry for yourself, it's advisable to focus on the positives referred to in this book and not to reflect on any setbacks from the day before or negative feelings that may appear as a result of sleep deprivation.

Zimmer

---◆---

In the very early stages, I would have been completely lost without my Zimmer frame and I am still amazed at how such a lightweight piece of metal can take someone's full body weight. I am surprised they do not add vehicle reversing noises, indicators and even urinals, but perhaps this may take off in the future.

Naturally, the hospital wants you up on your feet and using crutches as soon as possible and I was not provided with a Zimmer to use at home, although I admit that I borrowed one shortly afterwards.

The effort of getting into and out of bed meant that I needed to lean on something and I also slept better knowing that I would not face such a challenge when I got up in the night, which initially was very often.

Appreciating that you need to use all your muscle groups as early as possible, I suggest you speak to your medical staff about this upon your release and follow up on any advice they may give you.

Wishing all my readers the very best of luck with their operations and I very much hope that you, or your loved one, will make a full and speedy recovery.

www.ingramcontent.com/pod-product-compliance
Lightning Source LLC
Chambersburg PA
CBHW060716030426
42337CB00017B/2886